HEALTH
IN
YOUR FINGERS

By

DR ARPITA SINGH

DEDICATED

FOR

GOOD HEALTH

CONTENTS

A. INTRODUCTION

B. HASTA MUDRAS

    1. Gyan mudra

    2. Pran mudra

    3. Vayu mudra

    4. Akash mudra

    5. Shunya mudra

    6. Prithvi mudra

    7. Surya mudra

    8. Varun mudra

    9. Jalodar nashak mudra

    10.   Apan mudra

    11.   Apanvayu mudra

    12.   Ling mudra

    13.   Sahaj Shankh mudra

    14.   Kamar-dard nashak mudra

    15.   Jod-dard nashak mudra

    16.   Mukul mudra

    17.   Meao mudra

A. INTRODUCTION

Most health disorders, whether on the physical, mental or the emotional level, develop from a lack of inner and outer repose and / or too much stress or worry. An illness in the body is always connected with thoughts and feelings that make people sick. Hasta mudras have the wonderful effect on the inner peace especially in combination with pranayama and meditation.

Hasta mudras are the holistic way of healing of major and minor ailments with minimal efforts. These can be used to cure the diseases by those who are sick and confined to their beds or who no longer have the strength to practice the physical exercises of yoga as well as by a healthy person for the prevention of the diseases.

Hasta mudra means a specific hand posture made by keeping the fingers and hands in a certain manner. Mudras engage certain areas of brain and / or soul and exercise a corresponding influence on them.

However, mudras are also effective on the physical level. A certain amount of time is required before healing takes place on every level. So, allow yourself the time, practice ardently and remain completely serene and confident while doing so. Then, the chances of healing will be the greatest.

While performing the hasta mudra, the pressure of the fingers should be very light and hands must be relaxed. Do the hasta mudra as properly/accurately as possible and the effect will appear in any case.

Hasta mudras can be performed at any time while lying, seated, standing or walking although best results are obtained when these are done with pranayama and meditation in a seated posture thinking about the benefits of mudra. Generally, a hasta mudra is performed for 45 minutes in one sitting or in 3 time periods of 15 minutes each per day.

Initially, you may get tired quickly but with time your hands will become more flexible, strong and sensitive. You will feel more refreshed and energetic too. Your hands, especially the fingers, will become increasingly sensitive and respond to the mudras much more quickly after they have been given some practice. What I mean to say is, if you need 15 minutes initially to feel the effect of a mudra, in time you will need only 5 minute for that. This is really a wonderful experience! However, even if you are confined to your bed then you have enough time and can make good use of it.

The effect of a mudra may be perceived immediately or only after a certain amount of time. One can feel warm, the sense of unwellness and pain fades away, mood is improved and mind is refreshed. But, exactly opposite may also occur when you start the practice of a mudra. One feels tired or starts to feel cold and shivers. This is also a positive sign of the effect.

Hasta mudra yoga is based on 5 elements theory which are Earth, Water, Fire, Air and Sky. According to Indian Yogis all bodies are a combination of thesr 5 elements. Any imbalance in any of these elements leads to a disease and by balancing them, we can get rid off the diseases. This is what hasta mudras do. They balance the 5 elements in the body and cure the disease.

Now, I will flash a light on a few Hasta mudras alongwith a list of common health problems which can be cured by practising these hasta mudras.

B. HASTA MUDRAS

1. GYAN mudra

How to perform?

Join the tips of thumb and index finger.

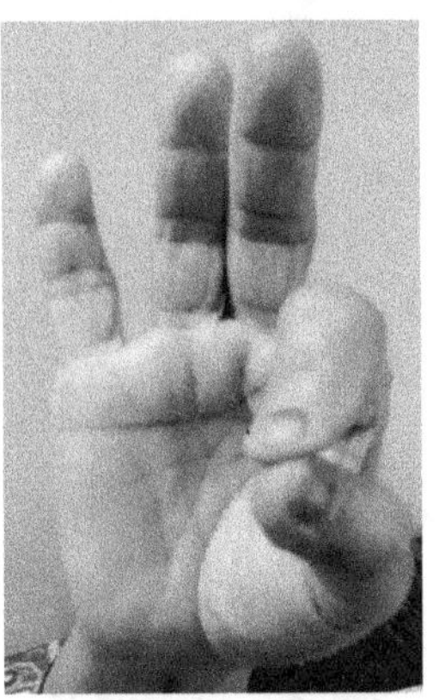

Benefits

This mudra is effective in case of weak memory, headaches, sleep disorders, tension, stress, depression, memory loss, forgetfulness, phobias, anxiety, anger, negative thoughts, weak nervous system, narcolepsy, mental and emotional weakness, Alzheimer's and hysteria, etc.

How to perform?

Join the tips of thumb, ring and small fingers.

Benefits

This mudra is effective in case of eye problems, general weakness, deficiency of vitamins, pain in legs, cramps in muscles, weakness after operation and weak immunity, etc.

3. VAYU mudra

How to perform?

Place index finger tip at the base of thumb by pressing it lightly by thumb.

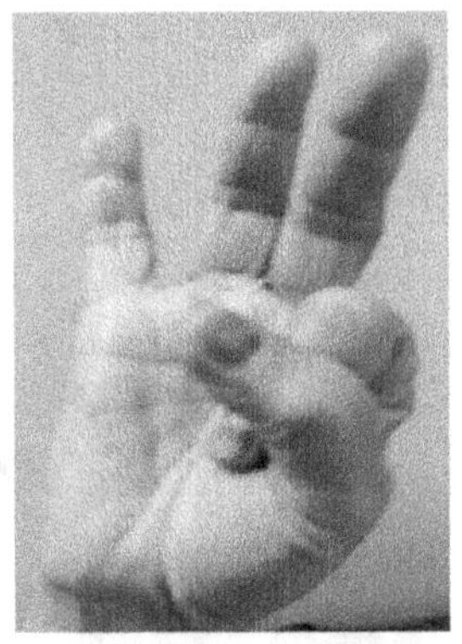

Benefits

This mudra is effective in case of pain in joints, viz., flatulence, gout, paralysis, sciatica, arthritis, Parkinson, spondiolytis, cramps in neck or back, pain in knee, cervical and back, etc.

4. AKASH mudra

How to perform?
Join the tips of thumb and middle finger.

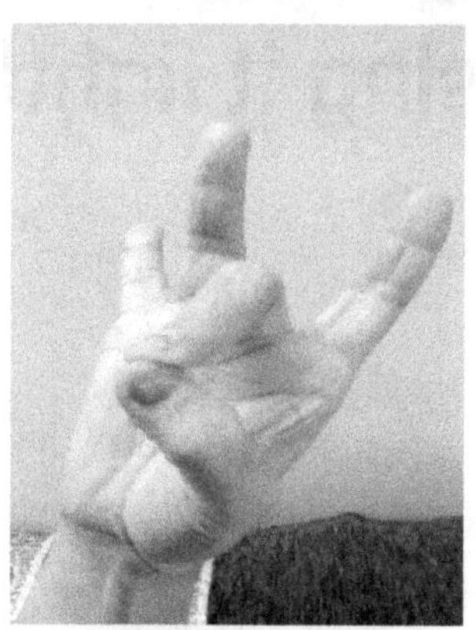

Benefits
This mudra is effective in case of bone weakness, jaw stiffness, osteoporosis and ear problems which can not be solved by Shunya mudra.

How to perform?

Place middle finger tip at the base of thumb by pressing it lightly by thumb.

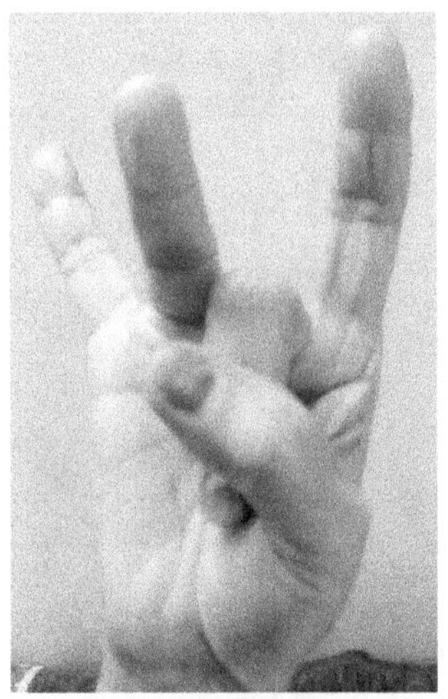

Benefits

This mudra is effective in case of ear pain, weak hearing, deafness, pus from ear, weak gums, throat problems, thyroid problems, ringing ears, dizziness while travelling and vertigo.

6. PRITHVI mudra

How to perform?
Join the tips of thumb and ring finger.

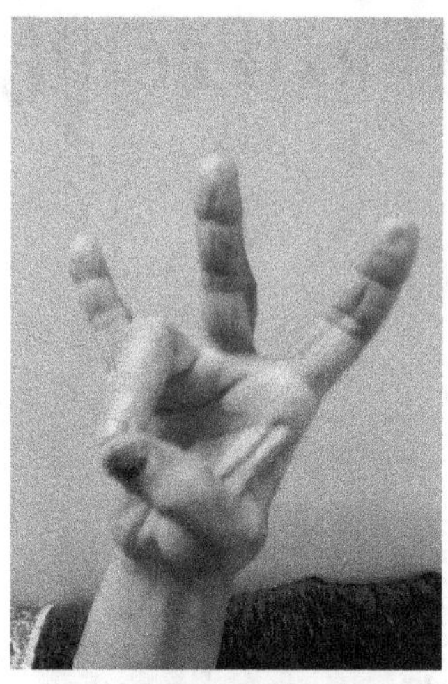

Benefits

This mudra is effective in case of thinness. Thin people can put on weight by this mudra. Also good for digestion.

7. SURYA mudra

How to perform?

Place ring finger tip at the base of thumb by pressing it lightly by thumb.

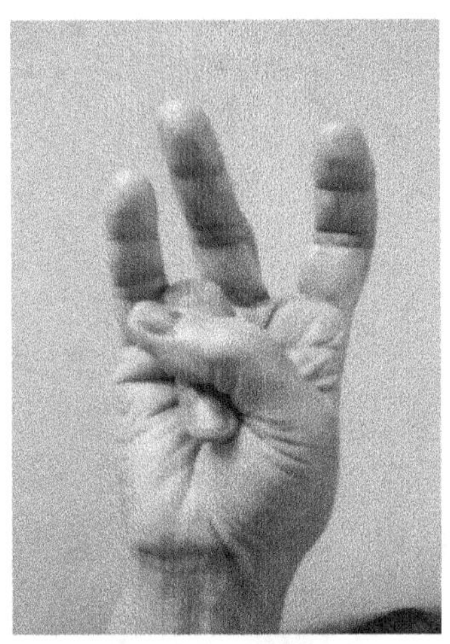

Benefits

This mudra is effective in case of excess fat and blood cholesterol, indigestion, diabetes and liver problems.

8. VARUN mudra

How to perform?
Join the tips of thumb and small finger.

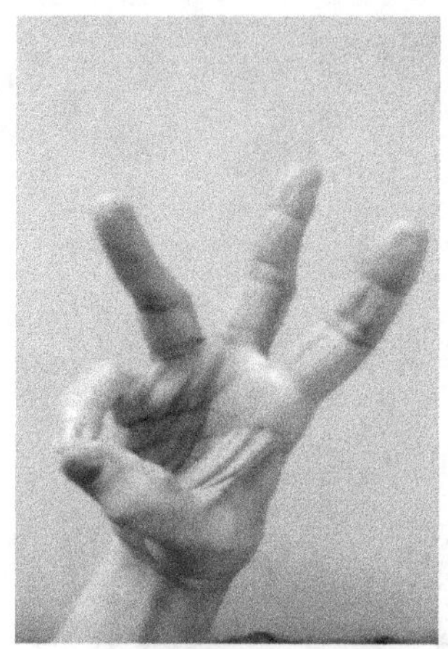

Benefits
This mudra is effective in case of skin problems, muscle shrinkage, eye hotness & gastroenteritis.

9. JALODAR NASHAK mudra

How to perform?
Place small finger tip at the base of thumb by pressing it lightly by thumb.

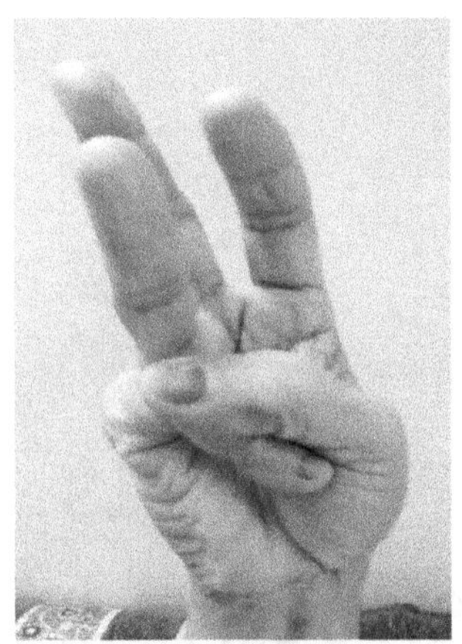

Benefits
This mudra is effective in case of excess of urine excretion.

10. APAN mudra

How to perform?
Join the tips of thumb, middle and ring fingers.

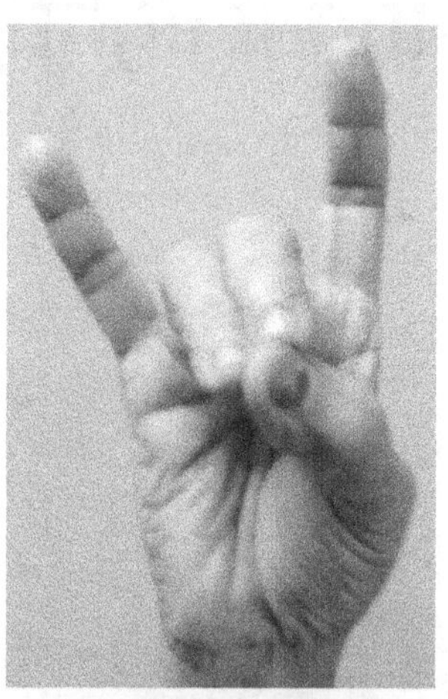

Benefits
This mudra is effective in case of piles, constipation, urine blockage, kidney diseases, flatulence, diabetes and teeth problems.

11. APANVAYU mudra

How to perform?

Place index finger at thumb base and join the tips of thumb, middle and ring fingers.

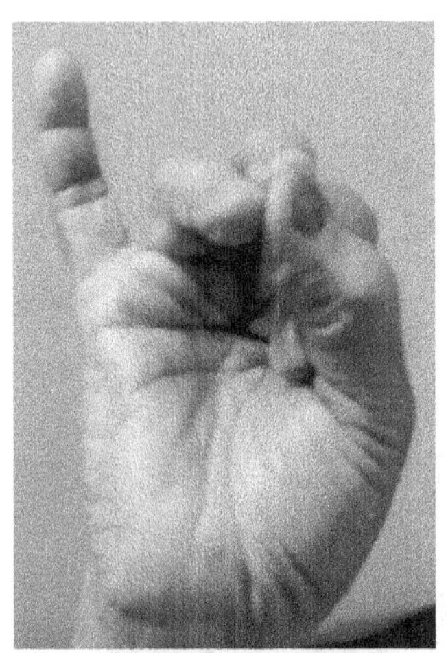

Benefits

This mudra is effective in case of heart attack, problems in breathing, emotional setbacks, anxiety, depression & acidity.

12. LING mudra

How to perform?

Interlock both hands with each other by keeping left thumb straight which will be in between index finger and thumb of right hand.

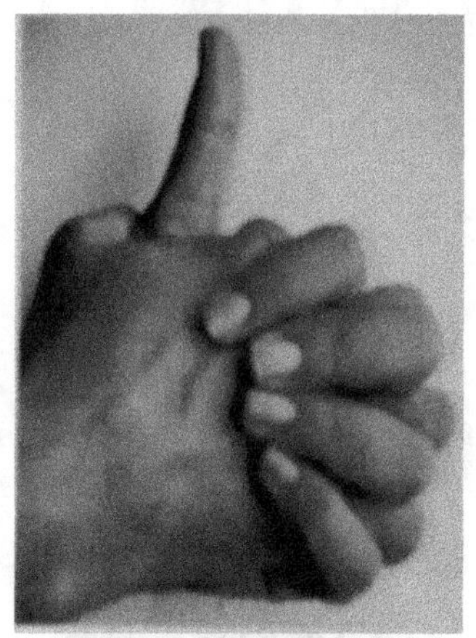

Benefits

This mudra is effective in case of cold, cough, when feeling extreme cold and low blood pressure.

13. SAHAJ SHANKH mudra

How to perform?

Interlock both hands with each other, keeping thumbs side by side.

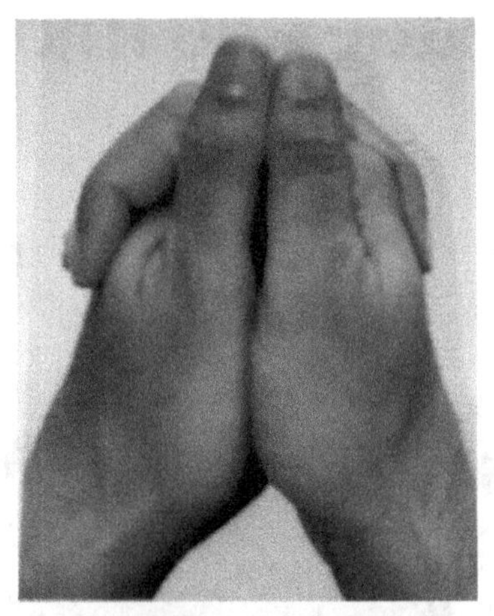

Benefits

This mudra is effective in case of thyroid problems, weak digestion, flatulence, stammering and speech problems.

14. KAMAR DARD NASHAK mudra

How to perform?

In <u>left hand,</u> place thumb on the nail of index finger and in <u>right hand</u>, join the tips of thumb, little and middle fingers.

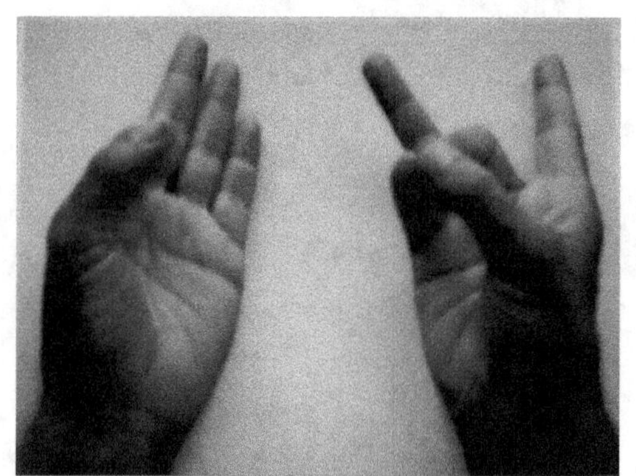

Benefits

This mudra is effective in case of back pain especially lower back pain, disc dislocation and slipped disc.

15. JOD DARD NASHAK mudra

How to perform?

Perform Akash mudra by left hand and Prithvi mudra by right hand.

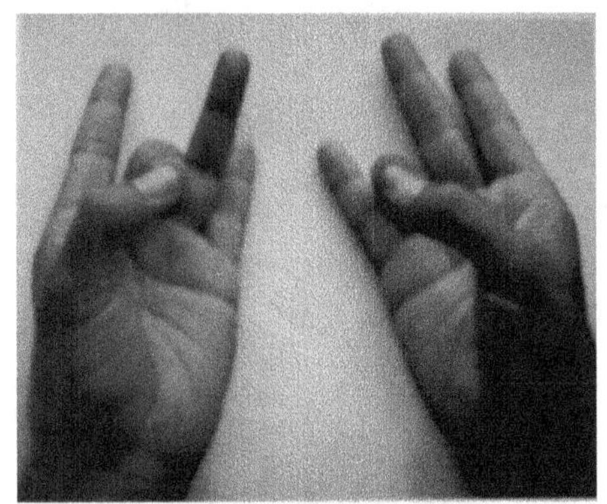

Benefits

This mudra is effective in case of pain in any joint in the body and arthritis.

16. MUKUL mudra

How to perform?
Join the tips of thumb and all fingers.

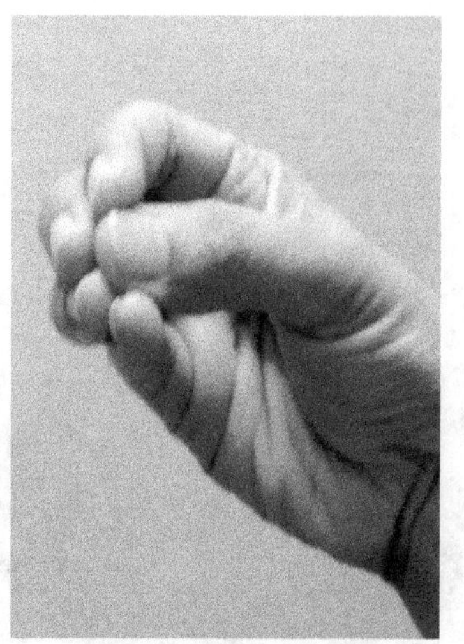

Benefits
This mudra is effective in case of weak immunity and general weakness.

17. MEAO mudra

How to perform?

Curl middle and ring fingers into the palm keeping other fingers normal.

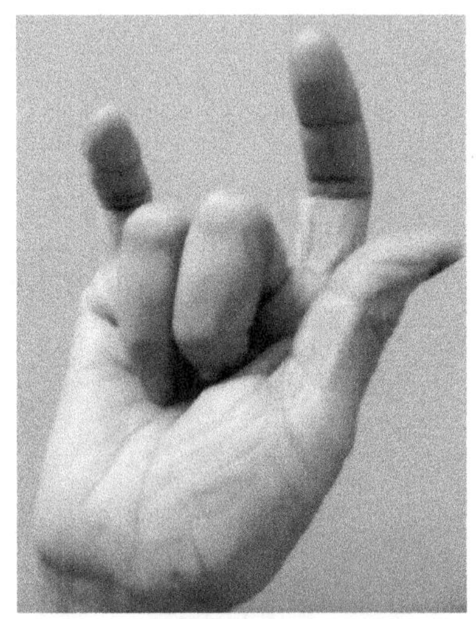

Benefits

This mudra is effective in case of both high and low blood pressure.

Read more....

1. Hasta-mudra Chikitsa Vigyan

   (ebook in Hindi)

2. Hasta mudra Chikitsa Vigyan

   (Paperback edition in Hindi, B/W),

3. Hasta mudra Chikitsa Vigyan

   (Paperback edition in Hindi, Full color),

4. HASTA MUDRA YOGA for EMERGENCY RELIEF

   (ebook in English)

5. Truthful experiments for health - KNEE PAIN (Part I)

   (ebook in English)

6. Truthful experiments for health - KNEE PAIN (Part II)

   (ebook in English)

7. Truthful experiments for health - GREEN BLOOD

(ebook in English)

8. Truthful experiments for health - CONSTIPATION

(ebook in English)